SILENT ECHOES

Navigating a World Without Sound

BY

SHAWN B. KATE

Table of Contents

Introduction: **Embracing the Silence**

It is simple to overlook the symphony of life that develops in stillness in a world that frequently resonates with the cacophony. However, it is in this stillness that we discover the amazing tales of deaf and mute youngsters, a world of grit, tenacity, and untapped potential.

This book takes the reader on a journey through the extraordinary lives of these young people. It makes an effort to shed light on their experiences, difficulties, and accomplishments as well as to recognize the beauty that resides in silence. We'll look at the power of assistive technology, the incredible connections within the deaf and mute community, and the language of the hands.

From the earliest stages of exploration through the inspiring times of accomplishment and self-expression. We will come across the families who provide unwavering support, the educators and professionals who offer guidance, and the advocates who stand up for the rights and possibilities of these children.

This book is mostly a tribute to the voices that flourish in absence of sound. It is a call to action to dismantle dices, dispel falsehoods, and celebrate the immense variety of human experience. We welcome you to accompany us on this excursion as we enter the world of deaf and silent children, hear about their experiences, and be moved by the melody that dwells within the silence.

Disclaimer

The content of this book, "Silent Echoes: Navigating the World Without Sounds," is intended for informational and educational purposes only. The author and publisher have made every effort to ensure the accuracy and reliability of the information presented within this book. However, it is important to note that the experiences and perspectives shared may not be universally applicable to every individual or situation.

In this book, Readers are encouraged to exercise their own judgment and seek appropriate professional advice when necessary. Readers are reminded that "Silent Echoes" is a work of non-fiction and should not be considered a substitute for professional advice or guidance. It is recommended that readers consult with relevant experts or specialists in the field when seeking information or support related to the topics covered in this book.

By reading this book, you acknowledge and agree to the terms of this disclaimer. Your use of the information contained herein is entirely at your own risk.

Chapter 1:   A Silent World

Imagine a world where a child's constant companion is stillness in a world that thrives on the symphony of sounds. This chapter embarks on a journey to explore the complex life that deaf and mute children live. It is a journey that immerses us in utter silence and awes us with how these kids manage in a soundless environment.

When seen through their eyes, silence, which is frequently taken for granted, transforms into a meaningful experience. It is a realm all its own, where connection, communication, and emotion all find particular expression. It is not only the absence of noise.

This chapter explores the inherent challenges that deaf and mute children confront, from their early stages of discovery to the myriad of challenges they face in a society that is built on speech and hearing. We'll talk about the loneliness and frustration that can come with living in silence as well as the incredible resiliency and persistence shown by these extraordinary kids.

We invite you to enter their world as we start our investigation, to observe the world quietly, and to travel with us as we attempt to understand and respect these extraordinary children's lives. By doing this, we can come to understand that this silence conceals a profound and lovely language that is just waiting to be revealed.

Chapter 2:   **The Language of Hands**

A new language emerges in a world devoid of spoken language. It is a language that defies aural limitations and relies on the dexterity of human hands and facial expressions. This chapter explores the fascinating topic of young deaf and mute people using sign language as a form of self-expression and communication.

A visual and expressive language, sign language—whether it's American Sign Language (ASL), British Sign Language (BSL), or one of the many other regional varieties—bridges the gap created by silence. It enables young infants to express their ideas, feelings and wants with astounding clarity. Similar to how spoken language combines words and syntax, sign language is composed of a complex and delicate system of hand movements, facial expressions, and body language.

We will demonstrate the beauty and power of sign language via sorrowful anecdotes and actual events. We will see the joy in a child's eyes as they learn their first signs, the conversations carried out with fast hand motions, and the sense of community and belonging created by shared gestures.

However, sign language is a gateway to culture and identity as well as a means of communication. We will look into the development of the distinctive culture and history of the deaf and mute group, which is largely based on the usage of sign language. This chapter allows you to immerse yourself in the world of hands that speak and, in doing so, to gain a deeper understanding of the incredible fortitude and inventiveness of these children as they make their way through a world where spoken language predominates.

We'll learn that the absence of sound need not be associated with a loss of voice as we investigate through the language of hands. Children who are deaf and quiet have a profound and elegant way of communicating, and in the stillness, they discover a special language that closely relates to their thoughts, feelings, and experiences.

Chapter 3: The Start of the Journey

Every journey starts with a single step, and for children who are deaf or mute, the path is filled with special challenges and triumphs. This chapter covers the initial stages of their journey, from the diagnosis of their illness to the crucial interventions that may determine their fate.

Parents and caregivers may start to pick up on signs that something is wrong during the calm period of infancy when chatting and cooing should fill the air. When a youngster doesn't respond to their voices, doesn't speak at all, or just stares at them with an unquenchable interest, these might be early signs that raise questions, fears, and frequently a whirlwind of emotions. We will discuss the delicate diagnosing procedure and the associated feelings. In this section, we'll look at how early intervention programs, audiologists, and healthcare professionals can all work together to prepare families for the challenges that lie ahead. This is a time of fear and uncertainty for many parents, but it is also a time of love and dedication to giving their child the best possible start in life.

The crucial choice of how to properly support a deaf and mute child's development marks the start of the trip.

While some parents choose hearing aids or cochlear implants to enable hearing, others may favor sign language as the main form of communication. We will examine the various paths that families choose as well as the factors that influence their decisions.

We will also look into the remarkable resilience of young children as they discover how to live in the world. Their intellectual and emotional development is greatly aided by early education and intervention programs. We'll hear stories of how young kids first encountered sign language, celebrated the success of their first words, and formed enduring bonds with their families and caregivers. While the road may be difficult as we pass through these early stages, it is also paved with love, hope, and the unwavering dedication of parents and other caregivers to providing the greatest future for their deaf and mute children.

Chapter 4:   A Family's Perspective

The journey through the life of a child who is deaf and mute is not their own; it is one they take with their families. This chapter focuses on the significant effects that a deaf and quiet child has on parents, siblings, and other members of the immediate family.

When parents discover their child is deaf and mute for the first time, it typically marks the start of an emotional rollercoaster. This chapter explores the range of feelings that are felt, from shock and sorrow through love, tenacity, and, in the end, acceptance. We'll talk about how to change expectations and goals as parents struggle with the realization that their child's life will not turn out the way they had hoped.

Siblings are important in the lives of a deaf and quiet youngster, too. We'll hear from brothers and sisters who had a sibling who had different opportunities and problems as they grew up. The connection between these siblings frequently develops into a source of assistance and comprehension, but it can also bring with it its challenges and traumas.

The entire family unit changes as it adapts to the needs and circumstances of the deaf and mute child. We'll talk about how families frequently act as educators, advocates, and sources of unending support. A family's support system benefits from the process of learning sign language and creating a positive communication environment. We'll also discuss the joys and triumphs of raising a deaf and mute child, including the first signs and words, shared laughing, and the numerous accomplishments that fill us with a deep sense of pride and satisfaction.

This chapter enables you to hear the voices and experiences of the families who set out on this extraordinary journey. The impact of a deaf and silent child extends well beyond the individual, changing the lives of those who walk by their side with unwavering support. It is a chapter of love, understanding, and resiliency.

Chapter 5:   **Education and Schooling**

A child's education is an essential component of their lives, and for a deaf and mute child, it takes on a special significance. This chapter explores the amazing young people's educational path, examining the value of inclusive education and specialized support in shaping their future.

In the classroom, children who are deaf or mute may encounter both opportunities and challenges. We'll discuss the benefits of inclusive education, which places students with a range of needs in the same classroom as their peers who can speak and hear. Inclusion gives a sense of belonging and normalcy in addition to offering a vibrant social atmosphere.

This chapter also emphasizes the importance of educators and teachers, who have a big impact on these kids' lives. We'll examine the instruction, methods, and tactics used to develop a welcoming and interesting learning environment. Deaf and mute kids' experiences in mainstream schools will be highlighted, showcasing their victories, friendships, and obstacles they overcame.

We'll delve into the function of specialist schools and programs created especially for deaf and mute pupils in addition to inclusive education. These facilities often offer a warm, welcoming atmosphere where teaching sign language is prioritized. We'll hear tales of artistic expression, intellectual and personal development, and the development of enduring friendships within these communities.

Additionally, technology and assistive devices have changed how deaf and mute student's study. We'll look at how people use things like hearing aids, cochlear implants, communication aids, and other gadgets to access spoken language and information.

We'll see as we proceed through this chapter that education for deaf and mute children encompasses not only the dissemination of knowledge but also a space for empowerment and self-discovery. It's a story of resiliency, creativity, and perseverance in the quest for knowledge, personal development, and a better future.

Chapter 6:   Overcoming Obstacles

A little child who is deaf and dumb travels through a world dominated by sound every day. This chapter explores the challenging process of overcoming societal stereotypes and prejudices to finally remove obstacles that prevent them from participating fully in society.

The challenges that deaf and mute children confront are numerous, ranging from myths and preconceptions to physical and mental challenges. We'll talk about why it's important to spread the word, push for reform, and disprove long-held myths.

Misperceptions frequently result in ignorance and, sometimes, discrimination. We will examine the difficulties and encounters faced by deaf and mute people as they interact with a society that usually fails to comprehend their distinctive perspectives. Their difficulties frequently include access issues, such as limitations on job opportunities, educational opportunities, and even recreational activities. This chapter highlights the necessity of greater equality and accessibility.

We'll also delve into the experiences of deaf and mute people who have turned to activism for both their own and other people's rights. Readers will be inspired and motivated by their accounts of bravery, persistence, and success in the face of adversity to take action for a more inclusive and equal society.

It takes all of us working together to remove these barriers, not only the deaf and mute community. To ensure that opportunities are available to everyone, regardless of their abilities, society as a whole must work to become more inclusive, to adopt the language of respect and understanding. This chapter seeks to further the belief that everyone should be permitted to live a life free from needless barriers and biases by igniting a larger discussion on the rights and potential of deaf and mute children and adults.

As we move through this chapter, we uncover tales of tenacity and advocacy, serving as a powerful reminder that a deaf and mute child has limitless potential as long as society acknowledges and respects their particular perspectives.

Chapter 7:   A World of Possibilities

Deaf and mute children navigate a world of remarkable possibilities and skills despite obstacles and constraints. In this chapter, we examine the diverse and fascinating array of skills, aspirations, and accomplishments that these kids bring to the fore. Just like any other child, every deaf and mute child has a distinct set of skills and passions. Young artists, aspiring scientists, eager athletes, and ambitious musicians will all be introduced to us; each will demonstrate the amazing possibilities that the world of quiet has.

The chapter serves as an example of how parental encouragement and support can help children develop these skills. It honors the accomplishments and aspirations of deaf and mute children who excel in a variety of fields, demonstrating that the lack of sound is in no way a barrier to excellence. Their success stories inspire us to think about what is possible and to realize that any child, regardless of talent, has the potential to achieve greatness.

This chapter also emphasizes how important mentors and role models are in giving these kids guidance and inspiration. These mentors frequently have similar experiences and serve as examples of accomplished goals.

Additionally, we'll look into how organizations and initiatives that support and promote the talents of people who are deaf or mute have an impact. These abilities are made more visible at art exhibitions, sporting events, and competitions, which reveals the beauty and depth of expression that lie within the silence.

This chapter aims to dispel stereotypes and forward the idea that deaf and mute children's skills are not constrained but rather an endless source of inspiration and surprise in a world where quiet is frequently misunderstood. It serves as a reminder that when children are given the support and opportunities they require, there are no limits to what they can accomplish.

As we sort through the abundance of options, we discover that there is a symphony of skills and dreams waiting to be heard, recognized, and valued in silence.

Chapter 8: Communication Beyond Words

Children who are deaf or silent have the innate potential to communicate in novel and inventive ways that surpass the limitations of spoken language. This chapter explores the fascinating world of assistive technologies as well as other forms of communication that support these kids' social interaction and self-expression.

When a child is classified as deaf and mute, a world of opportunities through assistive technology opens up. We'll examine the ground-breaking capabilities of cochlear implants and hearing aids, which can provide access to sound and spoken language. These tools give kids the chance to communicate with their hearing classmates and engage more fully in the audible world.

For many deaf and silent children, sign language, which was discussed in earlier chapters, continues to be a crucial part of communication. In this chapter, we'll learn more about the history of sign language and how it has helped the deaf and mute community communicate, express their feelings, and make friends.

We'll also explore the vast potential of alternative communication techniques including message boards, text-to-speech software, and graphic aids. young resources allow young kids a method to interact with the environment, express themselves, and engage in activities that go beyond spoken language.

The importance of educators, speech-language therapists, and assistive technology experts in facilitating the use of these tools is also emphasized in this chapter. These kids' knowledge gives them the ability to speak up, connecting them to a wider network of communication that goes beyond the limitations of silence.

We will reveal a universe of innovation, resiliency, and flexibility by exploring the various communication options. These children and the adults who help them are leading the charge to create a future in which communication has no bounds and the world is a more welcoming and inclusive place.

This chapter demonstrates the effectiveness of these techniques in assisting deaf and silent children in finding their voices and making connections with their environment. In the quiet, we discover a universe of novel and creative modes of communication.

Chapter 9: The Community of the Deaf and Mute

The deaf and mute community is a lively and resilient group that shares a unique connection within the rich tapestry of human experience. We'll delve into the sense of identity, support, and belonging that is woven into the fabric of this beautiful community in this chapter.

People who are deaf or mute frequently find comfort and understanding in a community of people who have similar circumstances. We'll examine the enduring friendships that are formed between group members throughout their formative years as well as the ongoing support and companionship that exists today.

As a common form of communication, sign language acts as a unifying factor for this community. It turns into a source of culture, pride, and identity. We'll go into the lengthy history of sign languages and discuss how important they have been in influencing the distinctive culture of the deaf and mute community.

We'll emphasize the importance of mentoring and support networks through the tales and experiences of community members. Young people who are deaf or mute frequently draw motivation and guidance from adults who have had a similar journey, supporting the idea that leading a fulfilling life is not only possible but highly cherished.

The importance of advocacy and group efforts within the deaf and mute population is also covered in this chapter. This organization catalyzes inclusion and change by promoting the rights of deaf and mute persons and bringing attention to the problems they face.

We'll also talk about the relevance of worldwide organizations and events that unite deaf and mute people from different backgrounds, as well as the deaf and mute community's global reach. For instance, the World Federation of the Deaf is an international spokesman for the rights and welfare of deaf people everywhere.

We will learn that inside silence, there lurks a rich and diverse tapestry of experiences, relationships, and collective power as we travel through the vibrant world of the deaf and mute people. It's a chapter that emphasizes the importance of common culture, identity, and activism while highlighting the notion that the relationships and understanding that develop in silence rather than what is said are what gives this group its strength.

Chapter 10: A Promising Future

A deaf and mute child's path has the potential of an inspiring future, despite its difficulties and unusual experiences. In this final chapter, we'll look at the triumphs, emancipation, and advocacy that show these exceptional kids' potential and accomplishments.

In the world of deaf and mute children, there are many triumphant stories. We'll meet people who have defied expectations, achieved academic success, followed fulfilling careers, and made advances in a variety of sectors. Their experiences serve as a testament to the incredible potential that deaf and mute people possess when given the right opportunities and assistance.

A symphony of victories is hidden in the stillness and is only waiting to be heard. This chapter emphasizes the empowerment and self-discovery that occur as these kids develop into tough, self-assured, and driven adults. Their path typically involves overcoming several challenges, but it also holds the promise of a life full of meaning, pleasure, and achievement.

We'll hear from activists and pioneers who have dedicated their professional lives to building a society that is more accepting and equitable for the deaf and mute population. These people push the bounds of what is conceivable, inspire change, and confront prejudices. Their work serves as a reminder that, with the right assistance, deaf and mute children can do anything.

The importance of ongoing education, assistance, and mentoring for deaf and mute children as they become adults is also emphasized in this chapter. Kids can develop into leaders, professionals, artists, and activists who make great contributions to society with the right tools and encouragement.

The message left behind as we come to the end of this book is strong: deaf and quiet youngsters have limitless potential. Their experiences are rich with triumphs, persistence, and the limitless potential of a life that thrives in solitude. Their stories inspire us to fight for change and to value the enormous variety of human experiences.

As a last thought, we are reminded that in the world of deaf and mute kids, silence is not a barrier; rather, it serves as a blank canvas on which the most amazing tales of success, empowerment, and optimism are painted.

Conclusion: Let's Celebrate Silence

We have delved into the unique world of deaf and mute children on the journey through the pages of this book. In this universe, being silent is not a sign of emptiness but rather a profound space where possibility, connection, and communication can flourish in extraordinary ways. We have witnessed these amazing children's struggles and triumphs, their tears and laughter, and their unwavering resiliency. The chapters have exposed the strength of the human spirit and the beauty that resides inside the stillness by sharing their experiences through exploration, education, communication, and community.

The experiences we've had shown us that embracing diversity and conquering obstacles go hand in hand. When given the right assistance, comprehension, and opportunities, children who are deaf or mute have limitless potential. We've found a symphony of talents, aspirations, and tales waiting to be acknowledged and appreciated in the silence. Young people who are deaf or mute live in a world of empowerment, self-discovery, and unwavering resilience.

As this chapter of the investigation comes to a close, we are left with the conviction that these children's, their families, and the larger community's lives are testaments to the resilience of people and the limitless potential of the human spirit.

The silence and the voices that abide in it are celebrated in this book. It's a call to action to smash down barriers, debunk falsehoods, and make sure that every child, no matter what their aptitude, receives the support they require to succeed. Let us take inspiration and the knowledge that beyond the quiet lies a world of beauty, power, and limitless possibilities with us as we part ways with these stories.